QUIZZES

1

What is the scientific study of the diagnosis, treatment, and prevention of diseases called?

2

What is the organ responsible for pumping blood throughout the body called?

3

What is the organ responsible for filtering waste products from the blood called?

4

What is the scientific study of the structure, function, and diseases of the human body called?

5

What is the organ responsible for producing hormones and regulating metabolism called?

6

What is the medical specialty that focuses on the diagnosis and treatment of diseases and disorders of the nervous system called?

7

What is the medical specialty that focuses on the diagnosis and treatment of diseases and disorders of the digestive system called?

8

What is the medical specialty that focuses on the diagnosis and treatment of diseases and disorders of the respiratory system called?

9

What is the medical specialty that focuses on the diagnosis and treatment of diseases and disorders of the urinary system called?

10

What is the medical specialty that focuses on the diagnosis and treatment of diseases and disorders of the circulatory system called?

11

What is the organ responsible for producing bile, which is necessary for the digestion of fats called?

12

What is the organ responsible for producing enzymes that help to break down food in the small intestine called?

13

What is the organ responsible for storing bile produced by the liver called?

14

What is the organ responsible for producing insulin, a hormone that helps regulate blood sugar levels called?

15

What is the organ responsible for producing hormones that regulate the menstrual cycle and fertility in women called?

16

What is the medical specialty that focuses on the diagnosis and treatment of diseases and disorders of the endocrine system called?

17

What is the medical specialty that focuses on the diagnosis and treatment of diseases and disorders of the reproductive system called?

18

What is the medical specialty that focuses on the diagnosis and treatment of diseases and disorders of the eyes called?

19

What is the medical specialty that focuses on the diagnosis and treatment of diseases and disorders of the ears, nose, and throat called?

20

What is the medical specialty that focuses on the diagnosis and treatment of diseases and disorders of the skin called?

21

What is the medical specialty that focuses on the diagnosis and treatment of diseases and disorders of the bones, joints, and muscles called?

22

What is the medical specialty that focuses on the diagnosis and treatment of diseases and disorders of the heart and blood vessels called?

23

What is the medical specialty that focuses on the diagnosis and treatment of diseases and disorders of the blood called?

24

What is the medical specialty that focuses on the diagnosis and treatment of diseases and disorders of the immune system called?

25

What is the medical specialty that focuses on the diagnosis and treatment of diseases and disorders of the brain and spinal cord called?

26

What is the medical specialty that focuses on the diagnosis and treatment of diseases and disorders of the kidneys called?

27

What is the medical specialty that focuses on the diagnosis and treatment of diseases and disorders of the liver called?

28

What is the medical specialty that focuses on the diagnosis and treatment of diseases and disorders of the pancreas called?

29

What is the medical specialty that focuses on the diagnosis and treatment of diseases and disorders of the thyroid gland called?

30

What is the medical specialty that focuses on the diag-nosis and treatment of diseases and disorders of the mouth, teeth, and gums called?

31

What is the medical specialty that focuses on the diagnosis and treatment of diseases and disorders of the throat, larynx, and pharynx called?

32

What is the medical specialty that focuses on the diagnosis and treatment of diseases and disorders of the nose and sinuses called?

33

What is the medical specialty that focuses on the diagnosis and treatment of diseases and disorders of the respiratory system, including the lungs, bronchi, and trachea called?

34

What is the medical specialty that focuses on the diagnosis and treatment of diseases and disorders of the urinary system, including the kidneys, bladder, and urethra called?

35

What is the medical specialty that focuses on the diagnosis and treatment of diseases and disorders of the female reproductive system, including the ovaries, uterus, and fallopian tubes called?

36

What is the medical specialty that focuses on the diagnosis and treatment of diseases and disorders of the male reproductive system, including the testes, prostate, and penis called?

37

What is the medical specialty that focuses on the diagnosis and treatment of diseases and disorders of the ears, including the auditory system and balance called?

38

What is the medical specialty that focuses on the diagnosis and treatment of diseases and disorders of the eyes, including the visual system and eye muscles called?

39

What is the medical specialty that focuses on the diagnosis and treatment of diseases and disorders of the skin, hair, and nails called?

40

What is the medical specialty that focuses on the diagnosis and treatment of diseases and disorders of the muscles, bones, and joints called?

41

What is the medical specialty that focuses on the diagnosis and treatment of diseases and disorders of the blood, including the production, circulation, and function of blood cells called?

42

What is the medical specialty that focuses on the diagnosis and treatment of diseases and disorders of the immune system, including allergies and auto-immune diseases called?

43

What is the medical specialty that focuses on the diagnosis and treatment of diseases and disorders of the endocrine system, including the glands that produce hormones called?

44

What is the medical specialty that focuses on the diagnosis and treatment of diseases and disorders of the digestive system, including the esophagus, stomach, intestines, and liver called?

45

What is the medical specialty that focuses on the diagnosis and treatment of diseases and disorders of the cardiovascular system, including the heart and blood vessels called?

46

What is the term for the abnormal accumulation of fluid in the body's tissues or cavities?

47

What is the term for the abnormal proliferation of cells, which can lead to the formation of a tumor?

48

What is the term for the abnormal production of red blood cells, which can lead to an excess of red blood cells in the body?

49

What is the term for the abnormal production of white blood cells, which can lead to an excess of white blood cells in the body?

50

What is the term for the abnormal production of platelets, which can lead to an excess of platelets in the body?

51

What is the term for a condition in which the body produces too much thyroid hormone, leading to an increase in metabolism and weight loss?

52

What is the term for a condition in which the body produces too little thyroid hormone, leading to a decrease in metabolism and weight gain?

53

What is the term for a condition in which the body produces too much insulin, leading to low blood sugar levels?

54

What is the term for a condition in which the body produces too little insulin, leading to high blood sugar levels?

55

What is the term for a condition in which the body produces too much cortisol, a hormone produced by the adrenal gland?

56

What is the average lifespan of a human heart cell?

57

How many bones are there in the human body?

58

What is the medical term for the condition of having too much sugar in the blood?

59

What is the function of the larynx in the human body?

60

How many chromosomes does a normal human cell contain?

61

What is the function of the pancreas in the human body?

62

What is the term for the medical condition in which the body's immune system attacks and destroys healthy body tissue?

63

What is the function of the spleen in the human body?

64

What is the term for the medical condition in which the body does not produce enough insulin?

65

What is the function of the thyroid gland in the human body?

66

What is the term for the medical condition in which the body produces too much thyroid hormone?

67

What is the function of the adrenal gland in the human body?

68

What is the term for the medical condition in which the body produces too much cortisol?

69

What is the function of the ovaries in the female body?

70

What is the term for the medical condition in which the body produces too much estrogen?

71

What is the function of the testes in the male body?

72

What is the term for the medical condition in which the body produces too much testosterone?

73

What is the function of the prostate gland in the male body?

74

What is the term for the medical condition in which the prostate gland becomes enlarged?

75

What is the function of the urethra in the human body?

76

What is the term for the medical condition in which the urethra becomes blocked or narrowed?

77

What is the function of the kidney in the human body?

78

What is the term for the medical condition in which the kidneys fail to properly filter waste from the blood?

79

What is the function of the liver in the human body?

80

What is the term for the medical condition in which the liver becomes damaged or scarred?

81

What is the function of the gallbladder in the human body?

82

What is the term for the medical condition in which the gallbladder becomes inflamed or infected?

83

What is the function of the small intestine in the human body?

84

What is the term for the medical condition in which the small intestine becomes inflamed or infected?

85

What is the function of the large intestine in the human body?

86

What is the term for the medical condition in which the large intestine becomes inflamed or infected?

87

What is the function of the esophagus in the human body?

88

What is the term for the medical condition in which the esophagus becomes narrowed or blocked?

89

What is the function of the stomach in the human body?

90

What is the term for the medical condition in which the stomach becomes inflamed or infected?

91

What is the function of the colon in the human body?

92

What is the term for the medical condition in which the colon becomes inflamed or infected?

93

What is the function of the rectum in the human body?

94

What is the term for the medical condition in which the rectum becomes inflamed or infected?

95

What is the function of the anus in the human body?

96

What is the term for the medical condition in which the anus becomes inflamed or infected?

97

What is the function of the respiratory system in the human body?

98

What is the term for the medical condition in which the airways become narrowed or obstructed, making it difficult to breathe?

99

What is the function of the circulatory system in the human body?

100

What is the term for the medical condition in which the blood vessels become narrowed or blocked, reducing blood flow to certain parts of the body?

101

What is the function of the nervous system in the human body?

102

What is the term for the medical condition in which the brain and spinal cord become damaged or diseased?

103

What is the function of the immune system in the human body?

104

What is the term for the medical condition in which the immune system becomes weakened or compromised, making the body more susceptible to infections and diseases?

105

What is the function of the endocrine system in the human body?

ANSWERS

1. Medicine
2. Heart
3. Kidneys
4. Anatomy
5. Pancreas
6. Neurology
7. Gastroenterology
8. Pulmonology
9. Urology
10. Cardiology
11. Liver
12. Pancreas
13. Gallbladder
14. Pancreas
15. Ovaries
16. Endocrinology
17. Gynecology or obstetrics (for females) and urology (for males)
18. Ophthalmology
19. Otolaryngology
20. Dermatology

21. Orthopedics
22. Cardiology
23. Hematology
24. Immunology
25. Neurology
26. Nephrology
27. Hepatology
28. Endocrinology
29. Endocrinology
30. Dentistry
31. Otolaryngology
32. Rhinology
33. Pulmonology
34. Urology
35. Gynecology
36. Urology
37. Otology
38. Ophthalmology
39. Dermatology
40. Orthopedics

41. Hematology
42. Immunology
43. Endocrinology
44. Gastroenterology
45. Cardiology
46. Edema
47. Neoplasia
48. Polycythemia
49. Leukocytosis
50. Thrombocytosis
51. Hyperthyroidism
52. Hypothyroidism
53. Hypoglycemia
54. Hyperglycemia
55. Cushing syndrome
56. The average lifespan of a human heart cell is about 70-80 years.
57. There are 206 bones in the human body.
58. The medical term for the condition of having too much sugar in the blood is hyperglycemia.
59. The larynx is responsible for producing sound through the movement of the vocal cords.
60. A normal human cell contains 46 chromosomes.

61. The pancreas is a gland that produces hormones such as insulin and glucagon, which help to regulate blood sugar levels. It also produces enzymes that help to digest food in the small intestine.
62. The term for the medical condition in which the body's immune system attacks and destroys healthy body tissue is autoimmune disease.
63. The spleen is a small organ that helps to filter the blood and remove old or damaged red blood cells. It also plays a role in the immune system by producing white blood cells and antibodies.
64. The term for the medical condition in which the body does not produce enough insulin is diabetes.
65. The thyroid gland is responsible for producing hormones that regulate metabolism and energy levels in the body.
66. The term for the medical condition in which the body produces too much thyroid hormone is hyper-thyroidism.
67. The adrenal gland is a small gland located on top of the kidneys. It produces hormones such as adrenaline and cortisol, which help to regulate the body's stress response and metabolism.

68. The term for the medical condition in which the body produces too much cortisol is Cushing's syndrome.
69. The ovaries are female reproductive organs that produce eggs and hormones such as estrogen and progesterone.
70. The term for the medical condition in which the body produces too much estrogen is estrogen dominance.
71. The testes are male reproductive organs that produce sperm and the hormone testosterone.
72. The term for the medical condition in which the body produces too much testosterone is hyperandrogenism.
73. The prostate gland is a gland located below the bladder in males. It produces fluids that help to nourish and protect sperm.
74. The term for the medical condition in which the prostate gland becomes enlarged is benign prostatic hyperplasia.
75. The urethra is a tube that carries urine out of the body from the bladder.

76. The term for the medical condition in which the urethra becomes blocked or narrowed is urethral stricture.
77. The kidneys are organs that filter waste and excess fluid from the blood and produce urine.
78. The term for the medical condition in which the kidneys fail to properly filter waste from the blood is kidney failure.
79. The liver is a large organ that performs a variety of functions, including filtering the blood, storing nutrients and energy, producing bile to help digest fats, and regulating the levels of various substances in the body.
80. The term for the medical condition in which the liver becomes damaged or scarred is liver disease.
81. The gallbladder is a small organ located under the liver that stores and releases bile, which helps to digest fats.
82. The term for the medical condition in which the gallbladder becomes inflamed or infected is cholecystitis.
83. The small intestine is a long tube that runs from the stomach to the large intestine. It absorbs nutrients from food and passes any remaining waste to the large intestine.
84. The term for the medical condition in which the small intestine becomes inflamed or infected is enteritis.
85. The large intestine is a tube that runs from the small intestine to the anus. It absorbs water and electrolytes from the remaining waste and forms it into stool.
86. The term for the medical condition in which the large intestine becomes inflamed or infected is colitis.
87. The esophagus is a tube that runs from the mouth to the stomach and carries food to the stomach for digestion.
88. The term for the medical condition in which the esophagus becomes narrowed or blocked is esophageal stricture.
89. The stomach is a muscular organ that mixes and grinds food and secretes acid and enzymes to help digest it.
90. The term for the medical condition in which the stomach becomes inflamed or infected is gastritis.

91. The colon is a long tube that runs from the small intestine to the rectum. It absorbs water and electrolytes from the remaining waste and forms it into stool.
92. The term for the medical condition in which the colon becomes inflamed or infected is colitis.
93. The rectum is the lower part of the large intestine that connects to the anus. It stores feces until they are ready to be eliminated from the body.
94. The term for the medical condition in which the rectum becomes inflamed or infected is proctitis.
95. The anus is the opening at the end of the digestive tract through which feces are eliminated from the body.
96. The term for the medical condition in which the anus becomes inflamed or infected is anitis.
97. The respiratory system is responsible for bringing oxygen into the body and removing carbon dioxide.
98. The term for the medical condition in which the airways become narrowed or obstructed, making it difficult to breathe, is asthma.
99. The circulatory system is responsible for pumping blood around the body and delivering oxygen and nutrients to the cells.
100. The term for the medical condition in which the blood vessels become narrowed or blocked, reducing blood flow to certain parts of the body, is arteriosclerosis.
101. The nervous system is responsible for coordinating and controlling the body's functions and responses to stimuli.
102. The term for the medical condition in which the brain and spinal cord become damaged or diseased is neurological disorder.
103. The immune system is responsible for protecting the body from infections and diseases.
104. The term for the medical condition in which the immune system becomes weakened or compromised, making the body more susceptible to infections and diseases, is immunodeficiency.
105. The endocrine system is responsible for producing and secreting hormones that regulate various functions in the body. hormones that regulate metabolism, stress response, and blood sugar levels. Other endocrine glands include the ovaries, testes, and pituitary gland, which produce hormones that regulate fertility and growth.

Printed in Great Britain
by Amazon

43558319R00020